50 Vegan Paleo Recipes

Disclaimer

No part of this eBook can be transmitted or reproduced in any form including print, electronic, photocopying, scanning, mechanical or recording without prior written permission from the author.

While the author has taken utmost efforts to ensure the accuracy of the written content, all readers are advised to follow information mentioned here at their own risk. The author cannot be held responsible for any personal or commercial damage caused by misinterpretation of information.
All information, ideas and guidelines presented here are for educational purposes only and readers are encouraged to seek professional advice when needed.

What Will You Find Inside?

This eBook contains 50 Vegan Paleo Recipes. It will help you cook Vegan-Paleo dishes for your everyday meal. The people who are looking for a healthy solution to their diet plans will find this eBook very beneficial.

So what if you are vegan? You can still follow a Paleo diet because it involves vegetables that are full of rich in nutrients that will keep you healthy as ever. All the recipes are strictly Vegan mixed with a Paleo diet routine.

You will find the following things in this eBook:

1. Introduction to Vegan-Paleo Diet
2. Variety of food that can be enjoyed in a Vegan-Paleo Diet
3. The benefits of following this diet
4. Strictly Vegan-Paleo recipes
5. Breakfast Recipes
6. Lunch Recipes
7. Dinner Recipes
8. Dessert Recipes

This report will help you learn about Vegan-Paleo recipes. By the end of this eBook, I promise you will be able to make Vegan-Paleo Recipes in every meal of the day. These recipes will be nutrient and protein rich that will surely provide you with proper nourishment.

Table Of Contents

Chapter I: Introduction

In the Old Stone Age or the Paleolithic era, anthropologists discovered that at this time people were hunter-gatherers. The hunters hunted for the meat with the tools they made and improved while the gatherers rummaged for fruits or vegetables they found edible. A Paleo diet starts with this small history wherein it incorporates the eating style of a caveman. This particular diet strengthened them and fulfilled the needed nutrition and energy the body required to perform daily tasks. Hunters and gatherers were active people; their whole day was about physical exercise and finding food. They had to perform tough tasks in order to collect food. The diet that helped them stay healthy is simply called the Paleo diet today. The name 'Paleo' is derived from the era that these hunters and gatherers lived in.

A Vegan-Paleo diet does not include eggs, meat byproducts, processed oils and dairy products. A vegan diet incorporates fruits and vegetables. Meat is an important part of a Paleo Diet but for all the vegetable lovers, Vegan-Paleo diet came into being. This diet is not less Paleo; it is as effective as a regular Paleo diet.

A Paleo diet focuses mainly on using whole and unprocessed food. It is highly encouraged in a Paleo diet plan to that no ingredient with artificial flavor will be added to the food. It is the healthiest diet plan and involves only pure food. Whoever follows a Paleo diet gets to avoid toxins from today's big production companies or farms such as genetically modified food. This diet will allow an intake of nutrients with less toxicity, which makes them healthier.

What Does A Vegan Paleo Diet Include?

Vegan Paleo diet is almost like a Paleo diet but with the meat removed. The idea is simple, to eat food that are unprocessed, chemical-free, toxic-free, sugar-free, salt free, dairy-free, and grain-free. There have been many arguments on a Paleo Vegan diet because it does not involve any source of protein and fat needed for the body. Yes, meat is the best source of protein but being on a Paleo Vegan diet won't make you a protein deficient.

There are some Vegan ways to include proteins. Although some are not as rich in protein as meat, they still provide enough to keep you on track. For example, the spirulina, fresh water algae, contains 65-71 percent more complete protein compared to 26 percent that beef offers in a 100g serving. Read the list of protein rich vegan food sources that you can incorporate in you Paleo Vegan diet.

1. Almonds
2. Spinach
3. Eggplant
4. Hemp Seed
5. Avocado
6. Sweet Potatoes
7. Pistachios
8. Spirulina
9. Beets
10. Celery
11. Butternut Squash
12. Cabbage
13. Figs
14. Grapes
15. Green Onions
16. Lemon
17. Lime
18. Bananas
19. Carrots
20. Peppers (All Kinds)
21. Yam
22. Zucchini
23. Watermelon
24. Walnuts
25. Tangerine
26. Cauliflower

27. Brussels sprouts
28. Broccoli
29. Asparagus
30. Artichoke hearts
31. Strawberries
32. Raspberries
33. Plums
34. Pineapple Guava
35. Peaches
36. Parsley
37. Papaya
38. Oranges
39. Mango
40. Lychee
41. Stevia
42. Macadamia Nut
43. Pecans
44. Sunflower Seeds
45. Pumpkin Seeds
46. Pine Nuts
47. Olive oil
48. Macadamia Oil
49. Hazelnuts
50. Grass fed Butter
51. Almond butter
52. Coconut milk butter
53. Coconut oil
54. Cashews
55. Cantaloupe
56. Blueberries
57. Blackberries

58. Avocado Oil
59. Avocado
60. Apple
61. Acorn Squash
62. Almond and coconut flour
63. Nutritional yeast
64. Some salts like; Himalayan sea salt, kosher salt, or any sea salt can be used in Vegan Paleo diet but remember, not to use excess amount of it.

Food That You Cannot Eat In A Vegan Paleo Diet

We have discussed it earlier that a Vegan Paleo diet does not involve any type of meat. Although meat is Paleo friendly and actually the best source for protein and good fat, a vegan diet does not allow you to eat meat. For your convenience, we are also mentioning the list of food that you should, at all times, *AVOID* while following a Paleo Diet. Refer to the list below to find out which food is a big NO-NO for you.

1. Eggs
2. Artificial Sweeteners
3. Juices (processed)
4. Meats
5. Beans
6. Grains
7. Dairy Products
8. Soft Drinks
9. Salty Foods
10. Junk Food
11. Alcohol
12. Energy Drinks
13. Starchy Foods
14. Candies

Anything that has been artificially manufactured is strictly prohibited in a Paleo diet. If you are not sure about using a product and it's not on our list of food to avoid, then make sure it is not artificially or chemically prepared. If it is, then it must not be eaten while on a Paleo diet.

What Am I Gaining By Following A Vegan Paleo Diet?

Most people are concerned about the benefits that a Vegan Paleo diet can provide for them. It is important to know this is a diet that is healthy and rich in nutrients. You don't have to second-guess if this diet is healthy or not because it just looking through the ingredients list; you will surely know. This diet does not and should not harm you in any way; instead it is very healthy and keeps you safe from many health issues such as diabetes and obesity.

Being a vegan itself is very healthy and even better if you are incorporating it in your Paleo diet. This makes it ever more beneficial. Never think of following a Vegan Paleo diet to be useless, it brings about positive and noticeable change in your health.

You might have learned from many people telling you how a Vegan Paleo diet is protein deficient. We do agree that vegan diet does not involve protein and fat rich substances but there are some food sources purely vegan that have some amount of proteins.

Chapter II: Vegan Paleo Breakfast Recipes

Almond Flour Pancakes

Ingredients

Granulated stevia - 2 tbsp

Coconut oil - 2 tbsp

Unsweetened applesauce (homemade) - 1/4 cup

Sea salt - 1/2 tsp

Baking powder - 2 tsp

Almond flour - 1 1/4 cups

Water - 1/2 to 1 3/4 cups

Preparation

1. In a bowl, add all the dry ingredients and whisk.
2. In another bowl, mix together ½ cup of water, applesauce and coconut oil.
3. Add the dry ingredients into the applesauce bowl.
4. Stir and keep adding the remaining liquid in small quantity.
5. Stop stirring once the batter forms a thick consistency.
6. Now cook for 2-3 minutes on a pan.
7. Cook for 2-3 more minutes from the other side.
8. Make sure both sides turn golden brown.
9. That's when you will know that your pancakes are done.

Grapefruit Sunshine Juice

Ingredients

Medium sized carrots - 4

Raw maca powder - 1/4 tsp

Fresh ginger – ½ inch piece

Peeled grapefruit - 1

Preparation

1. Place all the ingredients except maca powder in a juicer and blend.

2. Pour the mixture into a glass when smooth.

1. Stir in maca powder.

Strawberry Stacked Pancakes

Ingredients

Coconut Milk - 3/4 cup

Almond flour - 1 cup and 1/4 cup

Pure maple syrup - 1 tbsp

Cinnamon - 1/4 tsp

Allspice - 1/4 tsp

Baking soda - 1/4 tsp

Pinch of kosher salt

Warm water - 3/4 cup

Nutmeg - 1/4 tsp

Pure vanilla extract - 1/2 tsp

Baking powder - 1 tsp

Coconut Oil – For frying

Unsweetened shredded coconut - 1/2 cup

Strawberry Banana Soft Serve:

Frozen banana - 1

Strawberries - 3

Preparation

1. Preheat oven to 250 °F and line it with a baking sheet.
2. In bowl, whisk together almond flour, coconut, baking powder, baking soda, spices, and salt.
3. In another bowl, whisk together coconut milk, vanilla, warm water, maple syrup.
4. Now add to the dry ingredients.
5. Whisk well and make sure the mixture is smooth.
6. Pour some coconut oil in a skillet over medium heat.
7. Pour ¼ cup of batter onto the pan for each pancake and with a spoon spread it in a circle.
8. Cook each side for 2-3 minutes or until golden brown.
9. Transfer the pancakes onto a baking sheet and place in the oven to keep them warm.

10. In a blender blend the frozen banana and strawberries to make the strawberry banana soft serve.
11. Slice 20 strawberries.
12. Stack up the pancakes with strawberry pieces between each pancake.
13. Scoop strawberry banana soft serve on top of the pancakes.
14. Drizzle with maple syrup.

Paleo Latte

Ingredients

Ground cinnamon - 2 tsp

Coconut oil - 1 tbsp

Ground cloves - ⅛ tsp

Pitted date - 1

Boiling water - ½ cup

Ground cardamom - ½ tsp

Preparation

1. In a blender, add all the ingredients and blend on high until the mixture is smooth and frothy.
2. Easy Paleo Latte is ready to be enjoyed.

Blueberry Muffins

Ingredients

Pure almond extract - 1/2 tsp

Almond flour - 1 and 3/4 cups

Pure maple syrup - 1/2 cup

Olive oil - 1/4 cup

Coconut milk - 1 cup

Ground flax seed - 1/4 cup

Pure vanilla extract - 1 tsp

Baking soda - 1 & 1/2 tsp

Kosher salt - 1/4 tsp

Fresh and sweet blueberries - 1 and 1/2 cup

Ground cinnamon - 1 tsp

Apple cider vinegar - 1 tbsp

For cinnamon topping:

Vegan butter - 2 tsp

Almond Flour - 2 tsp

Honey - 2 tbsp

A pinch of Himalayan sea salt

Cinnamon - 1 tsp

Preparation

1. Preheat oven to 350 °F.
2. Line a muffin tin with liners.
3. Now mix together, coconut milk and apple cider vinegar in a small bowl.
4. Set the mixture aside.
5. Whisk together ground flax, baking soda, almond flour, cinnamon, and salt in another bowl.
6. In a small bowl, whisk together olive oil, maple syrup, pure almond extract, and pure vanilla extract.
7. Add the wet ingredients into the dry ingredients bowl and mix well.
8. Add in the fresh blueberries and stir to combine.

9. Spoon the mixture into paper liners.

10. For the cinnamon topping, blend all the ingredients and pour on top of the muffin mixture.

11. Bake the muffins in the oven for about 20-25 minutes or until the muffins turn golden brown.

12. Cool the muffins 15 minutes before serving.

Fruit-Nut Paleo Cereal

Ingredients

Almond milk – quantity of your choice

Flax seeds - 1 tbsp

Raw nuts - ¼ cup

Hemp seeds - 1 tbsp

Strawberries - ½ to 1 cup

Chia seeds - 1 tbsp

Preparation

1. In a bowl, pour the nuts and seeds.
2. Wash and cut strawberries into pieces.
3. Add strawberries into the bowl.
4. Pour almond milk into the bowl.
5. Your cereal is ready to be eaten.

Pumpkin Pie Oatmeal with Pecans and Pumpkin Pie Squares

Ingredients

For Oatmeal:

Regular oats - 1/3 cup

Pinch of sea salt

Pure vanilla extract - 1/2 tsp

Pumpkin - 1/3-1/2 cup

Nutmeg - 1/8th tsp

Coconut milk - 1 cup

Cinnamon - 1/2 tsp

Chia seeds - 1/2 tbsp

Ginger - 1/4 tsp

For the topping:

Crumble of Pumpkin Butter Oat Square - 1/3

Pure maple syrup - 1 tbsp

Pinch of cinnamon

Chopped pecans - 1 tbsp

Almond milk - 1 tbsp

Almond butter - 1/2 tsp

Preparation

1. Heat the almond milk and oats over medium heat in a pot.
2. Let the mixture come to a boil.
3. Add the pumpkin and chia seeds and stir.
4. Heat for about 5-7 minutes over low heat.
5. Stir frequently.
6. Add the spices and vanilla extract to the pot.
7. Heat for 5-6 more minutes while stirring frequently.
8. Place in a bowl.
9. Now for the toppings add all the ingredients over the oatmeal.

Raw Buckwheat Porridge

Ingredients

For the Porridge:

Unsweetened vanilla almond milk – 1 1/2 cup

Raw maple syrup –1/4 cups

Cinnamon - 1 tsp

Pure vanilla extract - 1 tsp

Raw Buckwheat Groats, soaked overnight - 2 cups

Chia seeds - 2 tbsp

For Toppings:

Chocolate chips

Almond butter

Chopped almonds

Chopped or dry fruits – you can use any fruit you like (strawberries, banana, raisins, kiwi, etc.)

Preparation

1. Add 2 cups of raw buckwheat and 4 cups of water in a bowl and soak for at least an hour before starting making the porridge.
2. Soak dry and pass through the strainer.
3. In a blender, place buckwheat groats, vanilla almond milk, chia seeds and vanilla extract.
4. Blend until the mixture turns smooth.
5. Now add maple syrup and cinnamon according to your taste (1/4 cup is for 4 bowl serving).
6. Place the mixture in glass bowls.
7. Add chopped or dry fruits of your choice, chopped almonds, almond butter, and chocolate chips on top of the porridge.
8. Serve cold or heat it up.

Spinach Pancakes

Ingredients

Warm water - 1/2 cup & 1 tbsp

Baking powder - 1 tbsp

Fresh spinach - 3 cups

Almond flour - 2/3 cup

Freshly ground flax seed - 3 tbsp

Preparation

1. In a bowl, place flax seed with water and set aside in the refrigerator to form a gel.
2. Add spinach and flax gel into a blender and blend.
3. Add baking powder and almond flour and blend until smooth.
4. On a griddle, add ¼ cup of the batter and use the back of a spoon to make a circle.
5. Cook each side for 3-4 minutes.
6. Don't let the pancakes turn brown, keep them light green.

Paleo Baked Cauliflower Casserole

Ingredients

Thinly sliced green onions – 2

Large head of cauliflower - 1

Coconut oil – 1 to 2 tbsp

Splash of coconut milk

Garlic powder, salt & pepper – to taste

Pinch of ground nutmeg

Preparation

1. Preheat oven to 375 °F.
2. Cut cauliflower into small pieces and boil in water until soft.
3. Drain the cauliflower and place back into the pot.
4. Add coconut oil, coconut milk and cauliflower into the blender.
5. Blend until the cauliflower is smooth.
6. Season with salt, pepper, garlic powder and a pinch of nutmeg.
7. Heat the mixture over low heat in a pot for a minute.
8. Remove the pot from heat.
9. Now add sliced green onions (save some for the topping).
10. Spread the cauliflower mixture into two greased baking sheets.
11. Bake for 25 minutes.
12. Once done, top with sliced green onions.

Green Monster Drink

Ingredients

Unsweetened vanilla almond milk - ½ cup

Kale - 2 cups

Frozen pineapple - 1 cup

Peeled and cored cucumber - 1

Pear, fresh and ripe - 1

Chia seeds - ½ teaspoon

Kiwi slice – For presentation

Preparation

1. Add all the ingredients into a blender leaving chia seeds out.

2. Blend until smooth.

3. Pour the smoothie in a glass and sprinkle with chia seeds.

4. Cut one kiwi slice a little till the middle and place it on the glass mouth.

5. Add a straw and enjoy.

Vegan Coffee Cake

Ingredients

For the crumb topping:

Almond meal - ½ tbsp

Unsweetened shredded coconut - 1 tbsp

Pinch of sea salt

Stevia - ½ packet

Applesauce - 1 tsp

For the cake:

Cinnamon - 1/4 tsp

Water – 4 tbsp

Baking powder - 1/2 tsp

Applesauce - 1/4 cup

Coconut flour - 2 tbsp

Stevia – 1 to 2 packets

Flaxseed oil - 1 tbsp

Preparation

1. In a bowl, place all the cake ingredients and mix well.
2. Make sure the ingredients are completely combined.
3. Grease a microwave safe mug.
4. Pour the mixture into it and set aside.
5. In another bowl, mix all the ingredients of the crumb topping.
6. Mix until combined.
7. Once mixed, sprinkle it on top of the cake mixture in the mug.
8. Place the mug in microwave and let it cook for 2 minutes.
9. Every microwave has a different timing; so make sure you keep a close look at the cake.
10. Let it cool and enjoy.

Chapter III: Vegan Paleo Lunch Recipes

Paleo Pesto Mashed Potatoes

Ingredients

Splash of coconut cream

Coconut oil - 2 tbsp

Sea salt – to taste

Minced garlic - 2 cloves

Pesto – 4 to 6 tbsp

Peeled Sweet Potatoes – 6 to 8

Freshly ground black pepper – to taste

Preparation

1. Cut potatoes in small cubes.
2. Boil sweet potatoes in a large saucepan until soft.
3. Strain the potatoes.
4. Add coconut oil and minced garlic into the same saucepan and cook over low heat.
5. Let it simmer for a few minutes to induce the flavor of garlic properly.
6. Add the boiled potatoes into the saucepan and mash.
7. Now pour coconut cream into the potatoes.
8. When the potatoes are fully mashed, add in pesto.
9. Season with salt and pepper.

Paleo Vegetable Curry

Ingredients

Turmeric - 1 tsp

Sliced carrots - 3

Green beans - 200g

Olive oil - 2 tbsp

Cumin - 2 tbsp

Chopped tomatoes – 1 tin

Chopped cloves of garlic - 2

Chopped sweet potato – 1

Chopped zucchini - 3

Chopped onions – 2

Black pepper and fresh coriander for seasoning

Preparation

1. In a pan, pour olive oil and add onions to fry for 3 minutes.
2. Add chopped tomatoes, beans and carrots into the pan and stir.
3. Simmer over low heat.
4. Now add chopped sweet potato into the pan and cover it leaving a slight opening.
5. Cook for 30-35 minutes.
6. Let the vegetables turn soft.
7. Add cumin and herbs and let the flavors infuse.
8. Once the dish is done, season it with fresh coriander and black pepper.

Sesame Noodles

Ingredients

Red pepper flakes to taste

Sliced green onions - 3

Sesame oil - 1 tbsp

Garlic powder - 1 tsp

Sea Salt and pepper to taste

Sesame seeds - 2 tbsp

Medium spaghetti squash - 1

Coconut oil - 1 tbsp

Chopped cilantro - 1/3 cup

Coconut aminos - ¼ to 1/3 cup

Preparation

1. Cut the spaghetti squash in half.
2. Place the halves on a baking sheet and bake in the oven for about 45 minutes.
3. Make sure the squash is soft.
4. Place sesame seeds on a cooking tray and bake until they turn brown and smell toasty.
5. Use a fork to open squash strings and place them in a bowl.
6. In a pan, heat the coconut oil and the sesame oil.
7. Now add green onions to the pan and cook for a few seconds.
8. Add spaghetti squash to the pan.
9. Add the remaining ingredients into the pan.
10. Cook for a few minutes.
11. Don't overcook the squash; it will turn hard.

Fresh Paleo Vegetable Salad with Italian Seasoning

Ingredients

Cauliflower - 1

Green beans – 1 pound

Red bell pepper - 1

Small red onion - ½

Black olives - ½ cup

White vinegar - 2 tbsp

Extra-virgin olive oil - ½ cup

Minced cloves of garlic - 2

Freshly ground black pepper - ½ tsp

For Italian seasoning:

Basil - ½ tsp

Marjoram - ½ tsp

Oregano - ½ tsp

Rosemary - ½ tsp

Thyme - ½ tsp

Preparation

1. Trim the green beans and chop the cauliflower into small florets.
2. Add water in a large pot and let it boil.
3. Add cauliflower and green beans and let boil for 3 minutes.
4. Let them stay tender-crisp.
5. Drain the water.
6. Place the vegetables in a bowl and set aside to cool.
7. Cut the red pepper into small pieces and red onions into thin slices.
8. Cut the olives into slices.
9. Mix all the vegetables in a bowl.
10. For the Italian seasoning, add all the ingredients in a bowl and mix until well combined.
11. Whisk together the white vinegar, the garlic, olive oil, the black pepper and the Italian seasoning (1 tbsp).

12. Pour the dressing and mix well.

Sweet Potato Pasta

Ingredients

Sea salt to taste

Medium sweet potatoes – 2

Sage - 1 to 2 tbsp

Cinnamon - 1 tbsp

Grass fed butter - 2 tbsp

Preparation

1. Wash sweet potatoes and peel.
2. Slice the sweet potatoes into thin strips.
3. Cut strips into quarter inch thickness and set aside.
4. In a large pan, melt the grass fed butter over medium heat.
5. Place the sweet potato noodle strips into the pan.
6. Stir continuously until the potatoes are cooked through.
7. Add sage and cinnamon and mix well.
8. Plate out and enjoy.

Mushroom and Vegetable Stroganoff

Ingredients

Water – 1 cup

Raw cashews - ½ cup

Red pepper

 Himalayan salt – 1 tsp

Chipotle pepper 1/8 tsp

Peeled and pressed garlic cloves - 2

Onion - ½

Butternut squash - 1

Nutritional yeast - ¼ cup

Fresh Mushrooms - 1 pack

Black pepper - ¼ tsp

Asparagus tips - 1 bunch

Fresh Lemon juice – 2 tbsp

Divided olive oil – 2 tbsp

Preparation

1. Peel and remove ends of the butternut squash.
2. In a slicer, slice butternut squash into noodles.
3. In a pot add water and some salt.
4. Place the noodles in the pot and boil for 2-3 minutes.
5. Cover the pot for 5 minutes.
6. Drain the noodles.
7. Add cashews, water, 1 tbsp olive oil, lemon juice, and nutritional yeast in a blender.
8. Blend until a smooth mixture is formed and set aside.
9. Chop asparagus, mushrooms, pepper, onion and pressed garlic.
10. Heat 1 tbsp olive oil in a pan over medium heat.
11. Sauté chopped vegetables in the oil.
12. Let the sauce thicken and reduce.
13. Plate out the noodles and top with vegetables.

Cauliflower Couscous

Ingredients

Pinch of Himalayan sea salt - optional

Cauliflower - 1 head

Olive oil - 1 tbsp

Preparation

1. Cut cauliflower into florets.
2. Transfer it to your food processor.
3. You can do this in two batches.
4. Start blending until florets are broken down completely and form a couscous.
5. In a pan, pour a tbsp of olive oil over medium heat.
6. Add couscous to the pan and sprinkle with a pinch of salt (optional).
7. Cover the pan and cook for 5-8 minutes.
8. Transfer the couscous into a bowl once it turns tender.

Lime-Cilantro Cucumber Salad

Ingredients

Black pepper to taste

Himalayan sea salt - ½ tsp

Fresh lime juice (homemade) - 3 tbsp

Crushed red pepper - 1/4 tsp

Seeded and diced jalapeno - 1

Finely minced garlic - 2 cloves

Olive oil - 3 tbsp

Finely sliced cucumbers - 2

Minced cilantro - 4 tbsp

Preparation

1. Dice garlic and jalapeno and place in a bowl.
2. Add crushed red pepper, 3 tablespoons of fresh lime juice, salt and pepper.
3. Add 3 tablespoons of olive oil while whisking continuously.
4. Add the finely sliced cucumbers to the dressing and stir lightly.
5. Finely chop the cilantro and add to the bowl.
6. Combine the ingredients in the bowl.

Layered Vegan Sandwich

Ingredients

For the tomato hemp basil pesto:

Water - 2 tbsp

Freshly ground black pepper – to taste

Oil-packed sun-dried tomatoes - 1/4 cup

Fresh basil leaves - 1 cup

Hulled hemp seeds - 1/4 cup

Fresh lemon juice (homemade) - 2 tbsp

Fine grain sea salt - 1/4 tsp

Extra-virgin olive oil - 1-2 tbsp

Large garlic clove – 1

For the sandwich:

Thinly sliced avocado - 1/2

Sun-dried Tomato Hemp Basil Pesto - 2 tbsp

Hummus - 2 tbsp

Grain free bread (made from almond flour)

Thin tomato slices - 1-2

Lettuce

Kosher Salt & pepper – a pinch

Red pepper flakes – a pinch

Preparation

1. For the pesto, mince garlic in a blender.
2. Add the remaining ingredients to the blender and blend until smooth.
3. For the bread, toast the bread in a toaster.
4. Layer the bread with hummus and pesto.
5. On both the slices of the sandwich.
6. Now place avocado, tomato, and lettuce over it.
7. Sprinkle the vegetables with red pepper, salt and black pepper.
8. Put the bread slice over it and enjoy.

Paleo Vegetable Stew

Ingredients

Water - 1 1/2 cups

Fresh lemon juice (homemade) - 1 tbsp

Minced garlic - 1 tbsp

Kosher salt - 1 tsp

Cumin - 1 tsp

Pure tomato paste - 6oz (no sugar and salt added)

Large chopped onion - 1

Un-peeled and cubed medium zucchinis - 6

Paprika - 1 tsp

Olive oil - 2 tbsp

Un-peeled and cubed large eggplant – 1

Black pepper - 1/2 tsp

Large chopped bell peppers - 2

Preparation

1. Whisk together, water, lemon juice, tomato paste, salt, black pepper, paprika and cumin in a bowl.
2. Set aside.
3. In a large saucepan add olive oil and cook over medium heat.
4. Place the onions in the pan and let it cook for 3 minutes.
5. Now add garlic, eggplant and zucchini into the pan.
6. Cook and stir until golden brown.
7. Add the tomato mixture and the bell pepper.
8. Blend everything together with a spoon and let it boil.
9. Turn the heat down to low and cover the pan.
10. Cook for 30 minutes while stirring occasionally.
11. Remove from heat and let it cool.

Stir Fried Cauliflower Paleo Rice

Ingredients

Soy sauce - 1/2 tsp

Sea salt and ground pepper - to taste

Small chopped onion – 1

Green peas - 1 cup

Coconut oil – 4 tbsp

Sesame oil - 1/2 tsp

Peeled and chopped carrots - 4

Chopped garlic - 2 tbsp

Cauliflower – 1 head

Coconut aminos - 6 tbsp

Preparation

1. Place the cauliflower florets in a blender and blend until finely crushed or rice sized.
2. Heat a pan over medium heat.
3. Add 2 tbsp of coconut oil and melt.
4. Add carrots, onions, and garlic into the pan and cook for 2-3 minutes.
5. Add peas and cook for another minute.
6. Sprinkle sea salt and pepper on top.
7. Remove from heat and set aside t cool it down.
8. Heat the remaining 2 tbsp of coconut oil in a pan over medium heat.
9. Add the cauliflower rice into the pan.
10. Toss in the oil.
11. Cook the rice for 5-8 minutes and stir constantly, so that the rice becomes golden brown.
12. Add the vegetables into the pan.
13. Stir and combine.
14. Now add sesame oil, soy sauce, coconut aminos and some additional sea salt and pepper to taste.

Chapter IV: Vegan Paleo Dinner Recipes

Spicy Tomato Soup

Ingredients

Water - 5 1/2 cups

Ripe tomatoes - 1 3/4 pounds

Olive oil - 2 tbsp

Ground coriander - 1/2 tsp

Mustard seeds - 1 tsp

Kosher salt to taste

Dried red chilies – 2

Turmeric - 1/4 tsp

Ground cumin - 1 tsp

Finely chopped medium onion - 1

Preparation

1. Peel and chop the tomatoes.
2. In a medium saucepan, heat olive oil.
3. Add the mustard seeds to the pan and cover the lid.
4. Let it cook until the seeds start to pop.
5. Turn the heat down to low and add onions.
6. Cook onions while stirring until they turn soft.
7. Now add cumin, turmeric, coriander and chilies to the saucepan.
8. Cook for about a minute and stir.
9. Add tomatoes and water into the saucepan.
10. Sprinkle a little kosher salt and leave it to boil.
11. Simmer the soup for about 30 minutes.

Roasted Spaghetti Squash with Kale

Ingredients

Sea Salt And Pepper – to taste

Balsamic Vinegar - 1 tsp

Spaghetti Squash - 1 whole

Kale - 2 bunches (stalks removed and torn into pieces)

Olive Oil – to taste

Chili Powder - 1/2 tsp

Diced onion - 1/2

Preparation

1. Preheat oven to 350 °F.
2. Cut down the spaghetti squash from the middle (length wise).
3. Spoon out the seeds and the pulp and discard.
4. Now place the squash on a large baking tray with the flat side up.
5. Cover the cut surface with olive oil.
6. Place it in the oven for 1 hour or until the squash is soft.
7. In a pan sauté the kale in olive oil.
8. In a pan heat olive oil and add onions.
9. Cook for 3-4 minutes or until the onions start turning golden.
10. Add kale, salt and pepper and stir until the onions are golden (for about 5 minutes).
11. Set aside.
12. Pull out the squash from the oven and scrape the soft squash from the shell using a fork.
13. Transfer the squash to a bowl.
14. Mix 1 tbsp of olive oil and balsamic vinegar in a small bowl.
15. Add into the squash.
16. Sprinkle salt, pepper and chili powder.
17. Toss to combine.
18. Sprinkle the top with sautéed kale and serve.

Layered Ratatouille

Ingredients

Zucchini - 1

Very thinly sliced garlic cloves – 2

Oregano - ¼ tsp

Divided olive oil - 2 tbsp

Tomato puree - 1 cup

Small eggplant – 1

Yellow squash - 1

Finely chopped onion - 1/2

Sea Salt and pepper – to taste

Few sprigs of fresh thyme

Crushed red pepper flakes - ¼ tsp

Long red bell pepper – 1

Preparation

1. Preheat oven to 375 °F.
2. In an oval baking dish, pour the tomato puree.
3. Add chopped onions and garlic cloves into the sauce.
4. Now stir in oregano, one tablespoon of the olive oil, crushed red pepper flakes.
5. Season the sauce generously with salt and pepper.
6. Remove the ends of eggplant, zucchini and yellow squash.
7. Remove the top and core of the red pepper.
8. Chop eggplant, zucchini, red pepper and yellow squash with a sharp knife.
9. Arrange prepared vegetable slices on top of the tomato sauce.
10. Starting from outside to the inside middle of the baking dish.
11. Covering the whole dish in layers.
12. Drizzle the remaining olive oil over the vegetables.
13. Sprinkle with salt and pepper.
14. Remove the leaves from the thyme sprig.
15. Add thyme leaves over the vegetables.
16. Cut a parchment paper to fit the baking dish and cover the dish with it.

17. Place in the oven and bake for 40-50 minutes until the vegetables have clearly cooked.

18. Make sure the vegetables are not wilted.

1. Pull out the dish from oven and enjoy.

Paleo Mediterranean Pizza

Ingredients

Italian eggplant – 2 (peeled, shredded & drained)

Ground flax seed – 2 tbsp + ¼ cup

Almond flour – 2 tbsp (blanched)

Olive oil – 1 tbsp

Sea salt – ½ tsp

Black pepper – ¼ tsp

Green and yellow zucchini – ½ cup (sliced)

Baby eggplant – ½ cup (sliced)

Graffiti eggplant – ½ cup (sliced)

Orange or yellow hothouse tomatoes – ½ cup (sliced)

Olive oil – 1 tbsp (for brushing)

Micro greens – 2 tbsp (to garnish)

Balsamic vinegar – 1 tbsp (to drizzle)

Instructions

1. Take a large bowl; mix together pepper, salt, oil, almond flour, ground flax seed and shredded eggplant.
2. Shape this mixture in a rectangle which is about ¼" thick. You can also use a rectangular baking tray to guide you with the shape.
3. Put parchment paper on an open sided cookie sheet and place the mixture on it.
4. Preheat your oven at 375°F.
5. Place the cookie sheet in the oven and start baking for at least 20 minutes.
6. Replace it from the oven, put a parchment paper over the crust and cover it with another cookie tray. Carefully flip the crust and remove the parchment paper from the top.
7. Place all the sliced vegetables on top and brush with olive oil. Season with salt and red pepper flakes if desired.
8. Place the sheet back in the oven and bake for 15 minutes.
9. Drizzle balsamic vinegar and top it with micro greens.
10. Serve hot.

Curry Tomato Soup with Zucchini Noodles

Ingredients

Zucchini – 4 (medium size)

Sweet Onion – 1 (sliced)

Olive Oil – 1 tbsp

Tomatoes – 3 cups

Vegetable Broth or Water – 2 cups

Red curry paste – 1 tbsp

Cumin – ¼ tsp

Fresh basil – ¼ cup

Red pepper flakes – ½ tsp

Salt – to taste

Unsweetened almond milk – 1 cup

Instructions

1. Heat oil in a pot, sauté onions for 5 minutes or till they soften.
2. Add salt, red pepper flakes, basil, red curry, water and tomatoes. Increase the heat and bring to boil.
3. Lower the heat once the mixture comes to a boil, cover the pot and let it simmer for 10 to 15 minutes.
4. For a creamy soup, add almond milk after 10 minutes and let it simmer for another 5 minutes.
5. When it is done, remove it from the stove and let it cool for a few minutes. Puree it in a food processor.
6. When it is time to serve, top with zucchini after warming it a little.
7. Top with almond milk, oregano, fresh basil and serve along with lime wedges.

Creamy Mushroom Soup

Ingredients

Unsalted Butter - ¼ cup

Fresh mushrooms - 2 pounds (sliced)

Salt – 1 pinch

Yellow Onion – 1 (diced)

All-Purpose Flour – 1 ½ tbsp

Fresh thyme – 6 sprigs

Garlic – 2 cloves (peeled)

Chicken Broth – 4 cups

Water – 1 cup

Whipping Cream – 1 cup

Black pepper and salt – a pinch

Fresh thyme leaves – 1 tsp

Instructions

1. In a pot, melt butter on high heat. Add mushrooms and salt. Cook the mushrooms till they juice and lower the heat.

2. Continue to cook on low heat till the juices of mushrooms evaporate and mushrooms become golden brown. This may take about 15 minutes.

3. Add onions with the mushrooms and cook till they become translucent and soft.

4. Add in flour and let it cook for 2 minutes while stirring. Take the thyme sprigs with a kitchen twine into a small bundle and put them into the mixture.

5. Add garlic, water and chicken stock. Simmer and cook for a minute. Remove the thyme.

6. Pour the soup into a blender and puree till it is thick and smooth.

7. After it is pureed, return the mixture in the pot and add in the cream.

8. Season with pepper and salt, garnish with a few mushroom slices and thyme leaves.

9. Serve.

Roasted Eggplant Salad

Ingredients

Eggplant – 1 (sliced)

Red onion – 1 (large cut in rounds)

Olive oil – as required

Avocado – 2 (halved, pitted and chopped)

Mustard – 1 tsp

Oregano leaves – 1 tbsp (chopped)

Honey – to taste

Pepper and salt – to taste

Lemon 1 (zest)

Parsley sprigs – as required

Instructions

1. Arrange the red onions and egg plant on a grill and brush them with oil. Cook and grill them till they are soft and slightly char.
2. Leave them to cool for a bit and chop them roughly.
3. Put them in a serving bowl with avocado.
4. Mix oregano, mustard and vinegar in a bowl. Include olive oil and honey. Blend well.
5. Season the mixture with pepper and salt.
6. Mix this dressing with eggplant and onion mixture. Toss well.
7. Top with parsley sprigs and lemon zest.

Super Soup

Ingredients

Oil – 2 tbsp

Onion – 2 (chopped)

Garlic – 5 cloves (minced)

Lentils – 16 oz

Water – 10 cups

Vegetable bouillon cubes – 2

Carrots – 3 (sliced)

Celery stalks – 3 (sliced)

Navy beans – 15 oz

Diced tomatoes – 15 oz

Brown rice – ¼ cup

Dried thyme – ½ tsp

Dried basil – ½ tsp

Oregano – a pinch

Pepper and salt – to taste

Instructions

1. In a large pot, heat oil on medium heat.
2. Sauté garlic and onion for 5 minutes or till they are tender.
3. Put in the rest of the ingredients.
4. Lower the heat and let it cook for almost 2 hours or till vegetables and rice are tender.
5. Serve hot.

Raw Veggie-Chili with Taco Nut

Ingredients

<u>For Chili</u>

Tomatoes – 3 cups

Red bell pepper – 1 (diced)

Celery stalk – 1 (diced)

Red or yellow onion – ½ (diced)

Zucchini – 1 (diced)

Corn off the cob – 1

Garlic – 3 cloves (minced)

Cilantro – to taste (chopped)

Chili powder – 2 tsp or to taste

Cumin – 1 tsp

Oregano – ¾ tsp

Sea salt – ¼ tsp

<u>Nut Meat</u>

Walnuts – 1 cup

Mushrooms – 1 cup

Cumin – 1 tbsp

Coriander – 2 tsp

Sea salt – ½ tsp

Instructions

<u>Vegetable Chili</u>

1. In a large bowl, add all the ingredients.
2. Put ½ of the mixture in a food processor and puree it.
3. Return the pureed mixture in the vegetables and toss.

<u>Nut Meat</u>

1. Pulse all ingredients in a food processor till they become crumbly.

<u>To Serve</u>

1. Put the vegetable chili in different bowls and sprinkle with nut meat.
2. Leave it for a few minutes at room temperature and serve.

Layered Vegetable Bake

Ingredients

Coconut Oil – 2 tsp

Zucchini – 1 (Sliced)

Eggplant – 1 (sliced)

Sweet potato – 1 (sliced)

Tomatoes – 5 (diced)

Water – 1 cup

Fresh Basil – ½ cup

Garlic – 1 Clove (Minced)

Coconut Sugar – a pinch

Pepper and salt – a pinch

Instructions

1. Preheat your oven at 180ºC and place baking paper on a baking dish.
2. Dust the eggplant and zucchini with salt. Leave it for 15 minutes to soften them up.
3. Take a non-stick pan and cook all the sliced vegetables for 3 minutes or till they soften.
4. Drain them on paper towel and set them aside.
5. Puree garlic, basil, water, tomatoes, pepper and salt in a blender.
6. Spoon this small amount of this mixture on the bottom of the baking dish.
7. Add a layer of zucchini, sweet potato and eggplant.
8. Top with sauce and repeat the layers till all sauce and vegetables are used up.
9. Add vegan cheese on top if required.
10. Put the dish in the oven and bake for 40 – 45 minutes or till the cheese (if used) has melted and the veggies are soft.

Spaghetti Squash Sesame Noodles with Edamame

Ingredients

Spaghetti Squash – 3 cups

Toasted Sesame Oil – 2 tbsp

Rice Wine Vinegar – 1 tbsp

Ground Ginger – a pinch

Garlic Powder – a pinch

Toasted Sesame Seeds – 2 tbsp

Green Onions – ¼ cup (diced)

Edamame – ¼ cup (cooked and shelled)

Cilantro – 9 sprigs

Soy Sauce – 3 tbsp

Instructions

1. Preheat your oven at 375 ºF.

2. Place the squash on a baking dish and bake for 45 minutes to an hour or till a paring knife can easily be inserted in.

3. Remove from oven and set aside to cool for 10 minutes.

4. Halve the squash lengthwise and scoop out all seeds.

5. Start scraping the squash with the help of a fork till all stringy spaghetti has been removed.

6. In a small bowl, add sesame seeds, garlic powder, ginger, vinegar, tamari and sesame oil.

7. Toss with spaghetti squash noodles and fold in edamame gently along with green onions.

8. Serve.

Black Bean Quinoa Sliders

Ingredients

Black Beans – 2 Cans (rinsed and drained)

Red Onion – 1 (diced)

Garlic – 3 Cloves (minced)

Button Mushrooms – 4 oz (diced)

Jalapeño – 1 (sliced)

Flax Meal – ¼ cup

Oat Bran – ½ cup

Tahini – ¼ cup

Quinoa – ¼ cup

Cilantro – 1/3 cup (chopped)

Cumin Seeds – 2 tsp (ground and toasted)

Coriander Seeds – 1 tsp (ground and toasted)

Pepper and Salt – to taste

Vegetable Oil – as required for frying

Instructions

1. In a pot, add ½ cup water with a pinch of salt and let it simmer.
2. When the water is simmering, add quinoa and let it cook till all water is absorbed.
3. Process tahini, jalapeño, mushrooms, garlic, onion and beans in a smooth mixture. Place it in a bowl.
4. Add in the rest of the ingredients and the cooked quinoa.
5. Mix everything well. Oat bran and flax will take a few minutes to fully absorb the liquid. So mix for a few minutes.
6. Place wax paper on a baking sheet and start forming your sliders. Place them on the sheet.
7. When all sliders are made, place the tray in a freezer for about 30 to 40 minutes.
8. In a heavy pan, heat vegetable oil and start placing the patties once it is hot.
9. Fry them for at least 4 minutes on each side.
10. Drain the sliders on a paper towel once they have fried.
11. Garnish with jalapeño, sliced onion and avocado.

Chapter V: Vegan Paleo Dessert Recipes

Apple Pie Quinoa Flake Muffins

Ingredients

Apple Sauce – ½ cup (unsweetened)

Flax gel – 2 tbsp

Quinoa Flakes – 1 cup

Ground Cinnamon – 1 tsp

Agave Syrup – 2 tbsp

Granny Smith Apple – 1 (diced)

Dried Almond Pulp – 2 tbsp (to garnish)

Instructions

1. Take two small ramekins and spray them with olive oil then set aside.
2. In a bowl, place flax gel, cinnamon, agave syrup and applesauce. Mix well
3. Include diced apple and quinoa flakes. Mix again.
4. Divide the mixture between the two ramekins while smoothening the top.
5. Top with dried almond pulp.
6. Put the ramekins in microwave for 3 minutes.
7. Let them cool for 3 minutes. Serve with natural yogurt.

Paleo Chocolate Mousse

Ingredients

Avocado – 1

Date Paste – ¼ cup

Unpasteurized Honey – 1 tbsp

Coconut milk – 1 cup

Organic Cacao Powder – ½ cup

Instant Coffee – 1 tsp

Ancho Chili powder – ¼ tsp

Himalayan salt – ¼ tsp

Pure Vanilla Extract – 1 tbsp

Instructions

1. Process coconut milk, honey, date paste and avocado in a blender till it become creamy and smooth.

2. Include vanilla, salt, chili powder, coffee and cacao powder. Process again till the mixture is blended well. Scrape sides to ensure all powder is mixed properly.

3. Pour the mixture in a bowl and start whisking for 5 minutes or till fluffy and light.

4. Divide the mixture between 4 to 6 dessert bowls.

5. Lightly dust chili powder or cacao powder on top and place in the refrigerator for 6 hours. It can be refrigerated for 2 days.

Vegan Pumpkin Banana Smoothie

Ingredients

Almond Milk – ¾ cup (unsweetened)

Crushed Ice – 1 cup

Frozen Banana – ½

Ground Flaxseed – 1 tsp

Pumpkin Puree – 1/3 cup

Maple Syrup or honey – 1½ tbsp

Ginger – ¼ tsp

Nutmeg – ¼ tsp

Cinnamon – ¼ tsp

Instructions

1. Put all the ingredients in a blender.
2. Mix well and pour into glasses.
3. Serve immediately.

Coconut Cream Pie with Chocolate Ganache

Ingredients

Chocolate Ganache

Dark Chocolate – 100 mg

Light Coconut Milk – 1/3 cup (unsweetened)

Almond Crust

Blanched Almond Meal – 1½ cups

Sea Salt – ¼ tsp

Ground Cinnamon – ¼ tsp

Baking Soda – ¼ tsp

Canola Oil – ¼ cup

Water – 1 tbsp

Cream Filling

Coconut Milk – 2 cans (unsweetened and unflavored)

Vanilla Stevia Drops – to taste

Vanilla Extract – as required

Topping

Coconut Flake – as required (unsweetened)

Instructions

Chocolate Ganache

1. In a microwave or a double boiler, melt the chocolate.
2. In a saucepan, pour in coconut milk and bring it to a boil.
3. Combing the chocolate and milk in a heat safe bowl and mix well.
4. Set aside.

Crust

1. Preheat your oven at 350 ºF.
2. Whisk together cinnamon, salt, baking soda and almond flour in a bowl. Ensure there are no lumps.
3. Include water and oil in the mixture with a spoon.
4. On a work surface, knead the dough till it is mixed properly.

5. Place the dough in a 9-inch pan making sure the sides are pressed up and it is evenly spread.
6. Transfer the dough on a baking sheet and bake for 10 minutes.
7. Brown the crust by broiling on low heat for 5 minutes.
8. Remove from oven and set aside to cool.

Cream Filling

1. Put the cans of coconut milk in the fridge overnight so that they are chilled when you start preparing this dish.
2. Open up the cans ensuring you don't shake them. Scoop the creamy thick part out and place it in a mixer bowl. Whip it on medium speed and gradually increase the speed to high. Whip for 5 minutes.
3. You will have thick whipped peaks.

Assembling

1. Place ganache on the bottom of the crust. Put it in the freezer for 15 minutes or till firm.
2. Over the ganache, place a layer of whipped cream.
3. Top with coconut flake.
4. Put the remaining ganache over the top and place in the refrigerator.
5. Serve chilled.

Vegan Chocolate Silk Pie

Ingredients

<u>For Crust</u>

Raw walnuts – 1½ cup raw walnuts

Cacao Powder – 1/3 cup (unsweetened)

Pitted dates – 1 cup (soaked in warm water for 10 minutes and drained)

<u>For Filling</u>

Silken Tofu – 12 oz (drained)

Semisweet Chocolate Chips – 1¾ cups (dairy-free)

Coconut Milk – ½ cup

Instructions

1. Start preparing the crust by pulsing cacao powder and walnuts in a blender till they become a fine meal.

2. Remove in a bowl and set aside.

3. Blend the soaked dates till the mixture is all sticky. Combine with the walnut and cacao powder mixture and blend again.

4. Lightly oil a glass pie pan, put a parchment paper on it and place this mixture in it. Cover the mixture with another parchment paper and press the mixture till a uniform crust is formed. Put the crust in the refrigerator.

5. In a double boiler, melt the chocolate chips or microwave them for 30 seconds.

6. Once the chips are melted, immediately place them in a blender and add coconut milk and tofu. Blend for 1 minute or till smooth.

7. Remove the crust from the fridge and pour in the chocolate chip mixture.

8. Cover the pan and place in the freezer till it sets.

9. Serve chilled with coconut whipped cream.

Paleo Lemon Bliss Bars

Ingredients

<u>For Crust</u>

Flax gel – 1 tbsp

Crushed Pecans – 1 cup

Coconut Oil – ½ cup

Almond Flour – 1 cup

Raw Honey – 3 tbsp

<u>For Lemon Topping:</u>

Lemon Juice – 1 cup

Flax gel – 6 tbsp

Raw Honey – ½ cup

Coconut Oil – ½ cup

Instructions

1. Put the pecans in a blender and pulse. Add in 1 tbsp of flax gel and blend.
2. Mix together coconut oil, honey, pecans and almond flour for the crust.
3. Spread the mixture on a pan, making sure it is even.
4. Place it in an oven and bake for 25 minutes at 350 ºF.
5. For the filling, mix together raw honey, flax gel and lemon juice in a pan and heat on medium heat.
6. Gradually add in the coconut oil. Stir continuously and once the mixture starts coating the back of the spoon, it means it is thickening.
7. Once it has thickened, spread it all over the crust.
8. Place the pan in the refrigerator for 2 to 3 hours.
9. Top with coconut shaving, cut into squares and serve chilled.

Vegan Strawberry Frozen Yogurt

Ingredients

Strawberries – 1 cup

Greek Style Yogurt – 2 cups

Raw Honey – 1/3 cup

Salt – a pinch

Instructions

1. Combine together honey, salt, yogurt and strawberries in a blender.
2. Mix well.
3. Place it in the refrigerator for 2 hours or more.
4. Churn the mixture in an electric ice cream maker.
5. Put in a freezer for 4 hours.
6. Serve chilled.

Paleo Chocolate Covered Mint Patties

Instructions

Mashed Potatoes – 1 cup

Salt – 1 tsp

Melted Butter – 2 tbsp

Peppermint Extract – 1 tsp

Confectioners' Sugar – 8 cups

Semisweet Chocolate – 8 squares (1 oz)

Shortening – 2 tbsp

Instructions

1. Combine peppermint extract, butter, salt and potatoes in a large bowl.
2. Start adding sugar to make it workable dough.
3. Start kneading the mixture and prepare small balls.
4. Flatten them in the shape of patties.
5. Place the patties on a wax paper and leave them overnight to dry.
6. Place shortening and chocolate in a bowl and microwave them till the melt and become smooth. Stir occasionally.
7. Sip the patties melted mixture and place them on wax paper.
8. Let them cool and serve.

Gluten-Free Paleo Cream Puffs

Ingredients

<u>For Pastry</u>

Milk – 1 cup

Unsalted butter – 4 tbsp

Kosher Salt – 1/8 tsp

Gluten Free Pastry Flour – 1 cup

Flax gel – 4 tbsp

<u>For Whipped Cream</u>

Heavy Whipping Cream – ¾ cup

Confectioners' Sugar – ¼ cup

Kosher Salt – 1/8 tsp

<u>Chocolate Drizzle</u>

Dark Chocolate – 4 oz (chopped)

Whipping Cream – ½ cup

Instructions

1. Start with the pastries, preheat your oven at 375°F.
2. Take two large rimmed baking sheets and place a parchment paper on them. Set aside.
3. In a heavy saucepan, heat salt, butter and milk. Let it cook till the butter melts and the mixture starts simmering.
4. Remove from heat and put in flour while stirring.
5. Place the pan again on heat, stir and cool till the mixture starts to pull away from sides and starts forming into a ball.
6. A thin layer will start forming at the bottom of the pan. Remove the pan and let it cool for 3 to 4 minutes.
7. Place half of this mixture in a blender and add in flax gel and then the rest of the mixture. Blend till the mixture becomes smooth.
8. Place this dough in a pastry bad with a large piping tip.
9. Pipe the dough in small mounds 1" apart on the baking sheet.
10. With wet fingers, smooth the top of the dough.

11. Put the sheet in the oven and bake for 10 minutes or till they turn pale golden.

12. Remove from the oven and immediately make a small slit on each side of all pastries with a sharp knife. This will allow some steam to escape.

13. Return the baking sheet in the oven and switch it off and open the door slightly. Leave them in the oven for 30 minutes.

14. Start working on the whipped cream while the pastries are drying.

15. In a large mixing bowl, add the cream and whip till soft peaks starts forming.

16. Include salt and sugar in the cream. Whip some more till it becomes stiff and glossy.

17. When the pastries are dried and cooled. Cut them in half horizontally.

18. Add in the whipped cream mixture on all the bottom halves then cover with the other halves.

19. For chocolate drizzle, cook the cream in a saucepan on medium heat till it starts to simmer.

20. In a heat proof bowl add the chocolate squares. Pour in the hot cream over them.

21. Start stirring till the chocolate melts and the mixture becomes smooth.

22. Pour the mixture over the pastries.

23. Serve chilled.

Vegan Blueberry Almond Tart

Ingredients

<u>For Crust</u>

Almond Meal – 2 cups

Maple Syrup – 3 tbsp

Canola Oil – 1 tbsp

Salt – 1/8 tsp

<u>For Filling</u>

Blueberry Juice – 1 cup

Fresh Blueberries – 2 cups

Cornstarch – 2 tbsp

Maple Syrup – 1/3 cup

Lemon Juice – 1 lemon

Slivered Almonds – ½ cup (toasted)

Directions

1. Preheat your oven at 350 °F.
2. Take a 9" tart pan and spray it with cooking spray. Set aside.
3. Mix together all the crust ingredients in a large bowl. Start combining it with your hands till the mixture is clumpy.
4. Pour this mixture into the tart pan and start pressing it down to create an even crust.
5. Place it in the oven for 20 minutes or till it turns golden brown.
6. In a bowl, mix together cornstarch and half of the blueberry juice. Whisk it well and set aside.
7. Take a saucepot and combine the rest of the blue berry juice, lemon juice, maple syrup and half of the blueberries. Cook and simmer the mixture for 3 minutes.
8. Carefully add in cornstarch and juice mixture while whisking continuously till the mixture thickens.
9. When the mixture thickens, put in the remaining blue berries and place it in the refrigerator for 2 hours.
10. Top with almond silver and press gently down before serving.

Vegan Mud Pie

Ingredients

Flour – 1½ cup

Sugar – 1 cup

Cocoa Powder – ¼ cup (unsweetened)

Baking Soda – 1 tsp

Salt – ½ tsp

Oil – 1/3 cup

Water – 1 cup

Vinegar – 1 tbsp

Vanilla Extract – 1 tsp

Instructions

1. Preheat your oven at 350 °F.
2. In a large bowl, add all the ingredients and mix well till it's smooth.
3. Take a 9" cake pan, line it with wax paper and pour all the mixture in.
4. Place it in the oven for 12 minutes.
5. Let it cool and cut in pieces.
6. Serve.

Vegan Orange and Almond Cake with Mascarpone

Ingredients

Oranges – 2

Caster Sugar – 250 gm

Flax gel – 6 tbsp

Almond Meal – 250 gm

Baking Powder – 1 tsp

Icing Sugar – as required

Mascarpone Cheese – 1 tub

Orange Zest – one orange

Crushed Almonds – as required

Instructions

1. After washing the oranges, place them in boiling water and cook for 2 hours.
2. Drain them and let them cool. Once the oranges are cool, puree them in a food processor.
3. Preheat your oven at 160 °C.
4. Butter a 20 cm cake tin and sprinkle with a little caster sugar.
5. In a bowl, mix together caster sugar and flax gel. Pour in the orange puree and baking powder and almond meal.
6. Pour this mixture in the cake tin and dust a little more caster sugar on top.
7. Put it in the oven for 1½ hours or till the top turns golden brown.
8. In a bowl combine orange zest and cheese. Pour the mixture over the cake.
9. Sprinkle some more caster sugar and almonds.
10. Serve.

Blood Orange Vegan Chia Pudding

Ingredients

Blood Orange Juice – 2 cups

Cashew Pieces – ½ cup (soaked overnight)

Honey – 1 tbsp

Chia Seeds – 3 tbsp

Coconut Sugar, Pomegranate Seeds and Blood Orange Segments – as required to garnish

Instructions

1. After draining the cashews, blend them in a food processor.
2. Pour in some of the orange juice slowly to thicken the cashew paste.
3. Blend for another 30 seconds to smooth the mixture.
4. Add in the rest of the orange juice.
5. In a nut milk bag, pour in the mixture and strain it. This will separate any cashew solids remaining in the mixture.
6. The mixture will be pink blood orange and creamy cashew milk.
7. Include chia seeds and mix well. Place it in the refrigerator.
8. After a few hours, take out the mixture and stir again then return it in the refrigerator. Leave overnight or for at least 9 hours.
9. Top with garnishing and serve shill.

Vegan Chocolate Cake Roll

Ingredients

<u>For Sponge Cake</u>

Energ Egg Replacer – ½ cup

Water – 1 cup

Sugar – 2/3 cup

Vanilla – 1 tsp

Flour – 1 cup

Cocoa Powder – 1/3 cup

Baking Powder – 1 teaspoon

<u>For Fluffy Coconut Crème</u>

Coconut Milk –1 can (chilled)

Maple Syrup – 2 tbsp

Vanilla – 2 tsp

<u>Fluffy Chocolate Butter Cream</u>

Coconut Milk – 1 can

Dates – 10 (pitted and soaked in water for 8 hours)

Cocoa Powder – ½ cup

Dark Chocolate – 6 oz (melted)

Instructions

<u>For Sponge Cake</u>

1. Preheat your oven at 300 °F.
2. Take a large bowl and add water and egg replacer. Mix well.
3. Whip the mixture with an electric mixer for 8 minutes on high till it gets fluffy.
4. Include sugar and whip some more for about 8 minutes till it double in volume.
5. Line a pan with parchment paper and oil it. Spray the sides as well.
6. Sift together baking powder, cocoa and flour. Add this in the whipped mixture.
7. On low speed, whip this mixture till it is combined properly.
8. Once done, spread the entire mixture on the pan and put it in the oven for 25 minutes.
9. Allow it to cool before taking it out of the pan.

For Fluffy Coconut Crème

1. Open the chilled coconut milk from the bottom and pour out the liquid. Place all the solids in a bowl and start whipping with an electric mixer.
2. Once stiff peaks start forming, include the vanilla and sweetener. Whisk some more till it combines. Place it in the refrigerator to chill.

Fluffy Chocolate Butter Cream

1. Mix together coconut milk, vanilla, dark chocolate, cocoa powder and soaked dates.
2. Whip till the mixture is smooth and creamy. Transfer in a container or bowl and place it in the refrigerator for several hours or till it becomes firm.
3. Pour this mixture in a large bowl and whisk with an electric mixer on high speed till the mixture becomes fluffy and light.

To Assemble

1. Flip out the sponge cake in a clean sheet of parchment. Peel of the parchment from the bottom.
2. Spread fluffy coconut crème over the top of the cake.
3. Start rolling the cake tightly from one end to the next using parchment paper as a guide.
4. Place the roll on serving platter and cut the roll diagonally.
5. Frost the cake roll with fluffy chocolate butter cream frosting.
6. Sprinkle powdered sugar on top.
7. Serve.

Vegan Chocolate Soufflés with Raspberry Sauce

Ingredients

Flax gel – 3 eggs

Yogurt – ¼ cup

Palm Oil Shortening – ¼

Vanilla Extract – 1 tsp (gluten free)

Arrowroot Flour – ½ cup

Maple Sugar – ½ cup

Cocoa Powder – 1/3 cup

Baking Powder – ½ tsp

Organic Raspberries – 1½ cup

Maple Syrup – ¼ cup

Instructions

1. Preheat your oven at 350 °F and prepare 2 ramekins by brushing them with butter or palm oil shortening.
2. Except for the raspberries and maple syrup, combine all the ingredients in a blender.
3. Blend at high speed till it becomes a frothy batter.
4. Divide the batter in the two ramekins.
5. Place in the oven and bake for 25 minutes.
6. While the soufflés are baking, take a saucepan and add maple syrup and raspberries in it.
7. Cook for 5 minutes on medium heat.
8. Put the mixture in a blender and blend till it reaches a sauce like consistency.
9. Once the soufflés are done, place them in a clean plate or leave them as they are. Top with the sauce and serve.

Conclusion

Eating a healthy vegan diet ensures that a healthy life. A Vegan-Paleo diet is a great way of ensuring that you and your family stay strong and fit throughout life. These 50 Vegan Paleo recipes will ensure that you have scrumptious dishes to eat and satisfy your cravings. These 50 Vegan Paleo recipes compiled in this book are all delicious and lip smacking and best of all are completely healthy.

SO don't wait up, start your Vegan Paleo eating today! Impress your friends and family with these healthy dishes while adding a bit of your own touch of creativity as well.